KITCHEN
Yoga

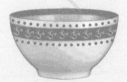

**Simple Home Practices
to Transform Mind, Body, and Life**

Melanie Salvatore-August · Illustrations by Rose Wright

yellow pear press

DISCARDED

Text copyright © 2015 by Melanie Salvatore-August.
Illustrations copyright © 2015 by Rose Wright.

All rights reserved. No part of this book may be reproduced in any form without written permission from the publisher.

ISBN: 978-0-9905370-1-4

Library of Congress Cataloging-in-Publication data available upon request.

Manufactured in China.

Design by Rose Wright.
This book has been set in Cronos Pro Light.

10 9 8 7 6 5 4 3 2 1

Yellow Pear Press, LLC

www.yellowpearpress.com

Distributed by Publishers Group West

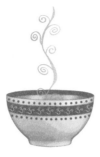

Table of Contents

Introduction

I love to love. My family is love, food is love, and yoga is love. The center of my home, where I enjoy much of this love, is my kitchen. It's the heart of the home and yoga is about keeping the heart healthy, both physically and emotionally. My yoga practice is about nourishment and using my highest intentions as food to fuel the vital energy of my ideal life.

The ancient practice of yoga is not just for the special few who have the time or luxury to devote hours each day to this once-secret health practice. Yoga—the art of uniting mind, body, and spirit—is actually a way of everyday living. It is a practice that creates the healthiest, happiest, most intentional person possible, and everyone has access. Change (whether physical or emotional) happens with small, sustainable actions throughout the day, and the practices I'm sharing are quick, doable, and enjoyable, yet powerful enough to shift your entire life for the better. The small home practices in Kitchen Yoga can align your heart's desires with your actions to strengthen your body and mind and lead to a happier, healthier life.

I have been practicing the simple yet profound practice of yoga since 1996, when I was introduced to it in New York City, I was a strung-out, anxious young woman who worried about everything and had the daily practice of mistreating her body. I overexercised, ate poorly, slept little, and cried a lot. Over the years, yoga taught me how to take care of my physical body and slowly, gently, started to challenge my unhealthy, harmful thoughts about myself. What I gradually discovered is that what one thinks, one experiences. That is the key to life because whatever you focus on will expand and become your reality. Yoga taught me to bring my deepest, kindest thoughts into alignment with my actions. It is from this personal experience that I share not only a strengthening and detoxing practice to be used throughout your day, but powerful intentions and affirmations to seed your mind with an abundance of healing thoughts. It is from these thoughts that you will find the energy of transformation. It is a winning recipe from the heart of your home—the kitchen—to nourish with love every aspect of your life.

CHAPTER 1

Cooking Up Love and Gratitude

I am abundant and thankful for a new day.

Fresh out of bed, I start my day in the kitchen—in my pajamas and a bit rumpled—where I consciously set the stage for my day. Just like the building of any structure, the stable foundation—the intentional beginning—is everything. That is why chapter one is the foundation of our practice. It is important to start here to build a stronger, happier you.

Our first practice in the morning is to become conscious that we can choose our thoughts and create our feelings, to detox the body of *ama* (toxins) accumulated in the night, and energize for the day.

Begin your day with a clear statement of love and gratitude such as, "I am abundant and thankful for a new day." What you think, you create, and believe it or not, our thoughts are our choice. We can actually program and reprogram our thoughts and choose those that will help

What you think, you create.

us be the healthiest, happiest beings we can be. Choose thoughts of love and gratitude, and they will energize you through any challenge or system of new growth, such as this new morning routine. When you are feeling doubt, fear, or lethargy, use the tool of repeating the positive statements associated with each pose described in this chapter to help change how you feel. And remember if you change your feelings, you will change your choices for the better. Use the affirmation, or *mantra* as it's called in yoga, in a relaxed state and simply repeat the mantra or affirmation I suggest with each pose (or another positive statement that you prefer) as you do the action sequences or any time you need a mental, emotional, or physical boost.

How we think and feel directly affects our breath, movement, and health. The simple, yet powerful tool of shifting your thinking is the perfect foundation to begin to detox, strengthen, and nourish your body. Let's begin the day.

Mountain Pose

(TADASANA)

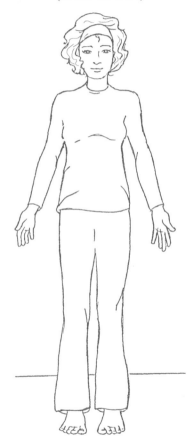

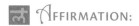 **A**FFIRMATION:

I am abundant and thankful for a new day.

Ingredients needed:

- Yoga block or tightly-rolled bath towel (optional)
- Slow even breaths, inhale equal to exhale

Stand with your feet hip-width apart with your feet parallel to each other (not turning out or in) with a yoga block in the thin position or tightly-rolled bath towel (optional) placed three inches below your groin and six inches above your knees and compressed between your thighs. Root down through your feet with even weight front and back, side to side, and then energize and lift your arches by engaging your thighs. Stand tall by aligning your feet, hips, and shoulders in one strong, steady stance with your chin parallel to the floor.

Mountain Pose is our template for balance and peaceful power. You will utilize the stance of Mountain Pose throughout your practice, and I invite you to explore it throughout your day whenever you are standing on both feet.

Gentle Low-Belly Lift

(MULABHANDA)

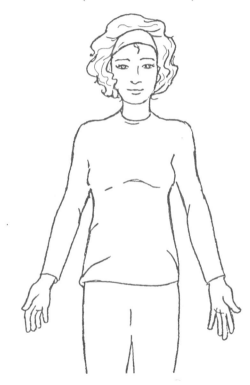

I am abundant and thankful for a new day.

Ingredients needed:

- Yoga block or tightly-rolled bath towel (optional)
- Tablespoon or teaspoon
- 16 ounces fresh, room-temperature water
- ¼ fresh lemon or 1 teaspoon apple cider vinegar (optional)
- Slow even breaths, inhale equal to exhale

While in Mountain Pose, stand at your sink and activate the lower belly region of the abdomen in an action similar to a kegel. This will support your low back, create greater stability for safe movement, as well as give you a feeling of calm groundedness, which is the way we want to start our day: intentional and balanced. From this point on, I will refer to this action as the Gentle Low-Belly Lift. Optionally, to create a stronger sensation of lift here, place a yoga block (in the thin position) or a rolled towel three inches down from the groin and six inches up from the knees, and gently squeeze your inner thighs while you do the following detox practices. These added props are not necessary but will help you have a more visceral feeling of that low-belly kegel lift that in yoga is referred to as mulabhandha.

Tongue Scraping
(IHIVA KRIYA)

Still in Tadasana, utilizing the Gentle Low-Belly Lift, we will scrape the tongue with a basic kitchen spoon to detox the body of built-up ama, or toxins, from the night. This practice will help boost your immunity and vitality, plus support fresher breath. Scrape from the upper back part of the tongue forward ten times. You will see a grayish-white film on the spoon, which is the sign that you are doing it correctly! Discard spoon for washing. Now that the nighttime toxins have been removed from your tongue, drink two 8-ounce glasses of fresh, room-temperature water. Do not sip this water but efficiently down it in a relaxed, sustainable manner. For an optional immune boost, add the juice from ¼ of a fresh lemon or 1 teaspoon of apple cider vinegar to the water (one or the other, but not both). Always scrape the tongue before drinking or eating anything for the day, because if you drink prior to scraping you will reassimilate the toxins from the night.

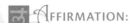 ## AFFIRMATION:

I am grounded and ready for greater abundance.

Ingredients needed:

- Wall, counter, or refrigerator handles
- Slow even breaths, inhale equal to exhale
- Gentle LowBelly Lift (see page 10)

Facing the wall, counter, or refrigerator handles, stand in Mountain Pose about six inches away from the surface. Touch your front hip points and then place your hands on the wall surface directly in line with your hip points, palms on the wall, with the heels of the palms in line with hip points and fingers pointing up toward the ceiling. With your hands pressing against the wall (don't move them!) back away from the wall until your arms are straight and your body is making a 90-degree L-shape (see illustration).

Next align your feet hip-width and parallel to each other with heels directly under hips. Soften and bend your knees to bring the spine in its natural curve and straight line. Press into your palms evenly as you stretch your buttocks away from the wall. With knees bent, breath five to ten slow, full breaths, and then slowly walk back toward the wall, counter, or refrigerator handles and resume Mountain Pose to reset and stabilize. Do two more rounds, beginning to lengthen through the back of the legs and stretching the spine in a slow, easy manner. Do not force the legs to straighten. Begin with your knees slightly bent or soft, and then slowly, as your muscles warm, you can build toward straighter legs. If your spine begins to round or there is any low-back discomfort as you straighten your legs, return to soft, bent knees.

Puppy Dog Pose

(MODIFIED ADHO MUKHA SVANASANA)

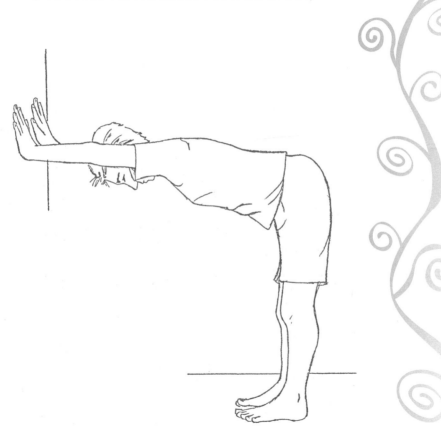

Mountain Twist

(PARIVRTTA TADASANA)

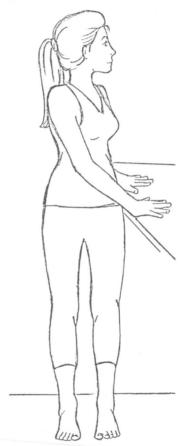

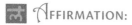 **AFFIRMATION:**

I am clear, light, and brimming with good health.

Ingredients needed:

- Wall, counter, or refrigerator handles
- Slow even breaths, inhale equal to exhale
- Inhale lengthen spine, exhale twist
- Gentle Low-Belly Lift (see page 10)

Stand tall in Mountain Pose with your right hip six to eight inches away from the wall, counter, or refrigerator handles. Align your body at a right angle to the surface with your feet parallel and hip-width apart. Activate your legs and belly to stabilize the pelvis. During this pose, the legs and pelvis will not move. Inhale and lift your sternum to lengthen your spine to stand as tall as possible and then exhale, draw your belly up and in, and turn just your chest to face the wall, counter, or refrigerator. Only the upper back and shoulders should be moving. Place your right palm on the surface, slightly below your right shoulder and with the elbow bent, and then lift your other hand into the same position on the left. Again inhale, stand tall, and then exhale and twist from the belly turning chest toward wall. Utilize a gentle pressing of the palms to the wall or counter to help facilitate a gentle twist in the upper back area. This will massage your spine and internal organs, facilitate detox, and relieve upper-back pain. Do this for five to seven breaths and then repeat on the other side, turning the opposite direction with your left hip, side, and pelvis perpendicular to the counter or wall. Do the same amount of breaths on each side.

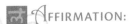

AFFIRMATION:

I am strong and can provide for myself.

Ingredients needed:

- Twisted dish towel (optional)
- Slow even breaths, inhale equal to exhale
- Gentle Low-Belly Lift (see page 10)

Step your feet one leg-length apart, turn out each leg from the hip socket, and align the center of your knee with the second toe of each foot. (If your knee is buckling in toward the midline instead of staying aligned with the foot, then turn your feet more midline and possibly shorten your stance slightly to align the knee with your second toe.) Bend your knees to a sustainable depth and lengthen your spine with your chest lifted, as in Mountain Pose. Stay in the pose for ten to fifteen breaths and then slowly straighten the legs, remaining in the initial pose. Take a few breaths and then slowly bend your knees and return to the full pose. Do this three times and sustainably increase the amount of breaths in each hold.

Once you are steady and can sustain the pose, take your hands behind your back and either clasp them by interlacing your fingers or take a towel between them to stretch the chest forward as well as release shoulder tension. Inhale, straighten your arms, and pull your chest open, bringing your upper back in toward the chest. If you clasp with your hands and your elbows resist straightening or your chest rounds closed, utilize a dish towel between the hands as a modified yoga strap and bring your hands as close together as you can, keeping this straight-arm, open-chest alignment. Do this additional stretch with each set of Standing High Squats or Goddess Pose.

Standing High Squat or Goddess Pose

(MODIFIED HIGH MALASANA)

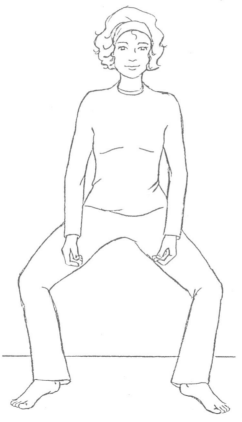

Soft-Kneed Wide-Leg Forward Fold

(MODIFIED PRASARITA PADOTTANASANA A)

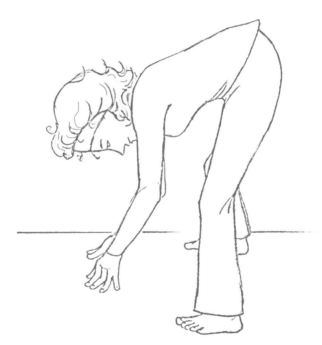

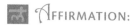
AFFIRMATION:

I am enough and can handle whatever transpires with ease.

Ingredients needed:

- Slow even breaths, inhale equal to exhale
- Gentle Low-Belly Lift (see page 10)

Stand with your feet one leg-distance apart and your feet facing forward and parallel to each other (not turned out or in). Standing tall as if you were in Mountain Pose, activate a slow, even breath and a Gentle Low-Belly Lift. With your hands on your hips, soften your knees and shift your weight slightly forward onto the balls of your feet, without lifting the heels. Inhale, lengthening your spine, and exhale very slowly beginning to fold forward from the pelvis while keeping your spine straight. Stop when your torso is parallel to the floor, bend your knees a little deeper, and pull your chest forward as you draw your shoulders away from your ears to further lengthen the spine. Keeping your knees bent, slowly lower your fingertips to the floor and breathe for five to ten breaths. Come up as slowly as possible, using the Gentle Low-Belly Lift, leading with your chest, and keeping your spine straight until you are back to a wide-stance Mountain Pose. Repeat up to three times, standing in Mountain Pose in between each repetition.

CHAPTER 2

Bathing in Creative Flow

I am the creator of my life.

The seed of intention

As a mother of three little boys I have become innovative on how to integrate my yoga practices throughout the day. Whether you're a parent, partner, or roommate, sometimes it may be difficult to get a moment alone. I find the bathroom a perfect place to catch a little time for myself to continue yogic grounding and detox practices. It is essential for manifesting radiant health to eliminate the physical, mental, and emotional toxins that build up from everyday life. These kriya (cleansing) techniques will take about fifteen to thirty minutes depending on how many options you apply. Aspire to do them daily as a part of your regular grooming. These practices will leave you detoxified, focused, and energized as you start your day.

As with any conscious action we take, the seed of intention is to be planted in love, gratitude, and abundance. Utilize the affirmations offered to weed out any thoughts of judgment, fear, or doubt that may reside and begin these practices with the acknowledgement that you are the creator of your experience. From a balanced, grounded place, you will intentionally create vibrant health and a peaceful, powerful mind.

is to be planted in love.

Proper Seat
(SEATED TADASANA)

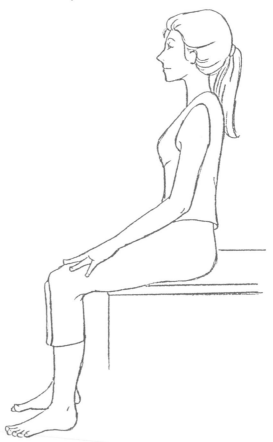

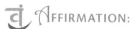

AFFIRMATION:

I am the designer of my day and my experience.

Ingredients needed:

- Area to sit (tub or stool)
- Slow even breaths, inhale equal to exhale
- Gentle Low-Belly Lift (see page 10)

Begin by sitting down on a steady surface, such as the side of the bathtub, the closed lid of the toilet, or a stool. Create a steady and even seat by making sure your sitting bones are evenly rooted to the seat surface. Align your feet hip-width apart and parallel, with your heels directly underneath your knees. Root into your feet and sitting bones evenly and rise up through the spine lifting the sternum up toward the ceiling. Draw the elbows underneath the shoulder joint and widen your collarbones to gently open the chest. Bring your chin parallel to the floor and settle your eyes on one point of focus nose height. Relax the entire face and create an even breath, inhale equal to exhale, with little to no pause.

ॐ Affirmation:

I am receptive and giving.

Ingredients needed:

- Proper Seat (see previous)
- Slow even breaths, inhale equal to exhale
- Gentle Low-Belly Lift (see page 10)

This pranayama (breath exercise) will slow your heart rate and relax your mind and body. It can be done anywhere at any time to reduce stress and increase clarity. It can be done either standing or sitting, but it is easiest to focus and feel when in a proper sitting position. From the Proper Seat position, with a straight spine and supported neck, shift from the pelvis forward, bringing lower belly onto the thighs. Slowly increase your inhale, making it conscious and deliberate while filling the belly until it opens to the side and all the way around to the low-back area below the bottom ribs. Slowly exhale in a deliberate action, creating an exhalation equal to the original inhalation (equal in timing and quality). Repeat for ten breaths and then very slowly return to an upright position. Remain still for thirty seconds, allowing the body to readjust and feel the effects of the practice. Repeat the series until feeling more centered, relaxed, and clear. Pranayama can be used anytime throughout the day when you might be experiencing stress.

Full and Complete
Balanced Breath
(PRANAYAMA)

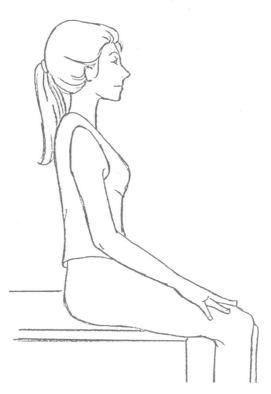

Easy Forward Fold
(UTTANASANA)

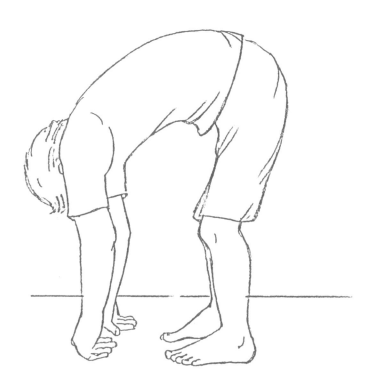

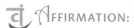 **AFFIRMATION:**

I am an artist of abundance.

Ingredients needed:

- Mountain Pose or Proper Seat

- Slow even breaths, inhale equal to exhale

- Gentle Low-Belly Lift (see page 10)

Begin by standing in Mountain Pose or Proper Seat with the feet hip-width apart and parallel to each other. Inhale and lengthen through the spine and, as you exhale, firm the belly and begin to fold from the hips. Gently bend both knees, keeping the knees aligned with the second toe and shifting the weight of the body slightly forward onto the balls of the feet. Release and hang the spine, head, and neck to release tension in the spine and gently stretch the back. Keep the knees bent and weight shifted slightly forward as you hang for five full and complete breaths, creating a pressure on the low belly with the top of the thighs to help press the breath into the side ribs and back body with each breath. When ready to ascend, press evenly into the feet, firm the core muscles, and slowly with a flat back come up halfway, pause for one breath to stabilize, and then on the next inhale, rise all the way to standing position. Stand still in Mountain Pose for a few breaths before either repeating uttanasana (up to three times) or moving on to the next practice. Choose the Proper Seat instead of Mountain Pose for this practice if more stability or support for the body is needed.

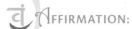

AFFIRMATION:

I let go of what no longer serves me.

Ingredients needed:

- Mountain Pose or Proper Seat
- 1 Tablespoon organic coconut oil or sesame oil
- Tissue for disposal of oil
- Timer (optional)
- Spoon (optional)
- Toothbrush / toothpaste
- Slow even breaths, inhale equal to exhale
- Gentle Low-Belly Lift (see page 10)

Stand in Mountain Pose or sit in Proper Seat to begin the process of removing bacteria and toxins from the mouth and body. Take a tablespoon of organic coconut or sesame oil and place it in your mouth. Do not swallow! Begin to swish the oil around the mouth and through the teeth. The first minute may be unappealing, but it will become easier with practice. Continue swishing and pulling the oil evenly throughout the entire mouth without swallowing for as long as possible (ideally up to twenty minutes). When you have finished, spit the oil into a tissue or directly into the garbage can but not into the sink or drain because these oils tend to thicken and will clog the pipes! After spitting, brush your teeth and tongue for two minutes and then swish your mouth with water to complete the practice.

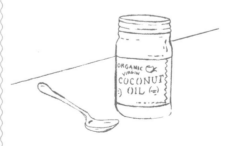

Detox Oil Swishing

(KAVALA GRAHA)

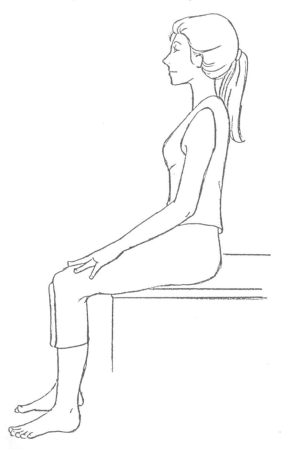

Detox Dry Brushing

(TVACHA KRIYA)

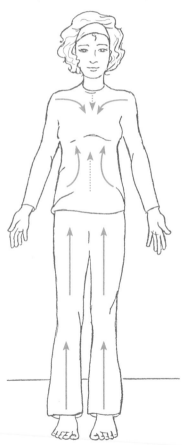

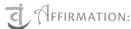

AFFIRMATION:

I release harmful, old habits and create powerful, positive, new ones.

Ingredients needed:

- Mountain Pose or Proper Seat
- Natural body brush (with a handle long enough to reach your back)
- Slow even breaths, inhale equal to exhale
- Gentle Low-Belly Lift (see page 10)

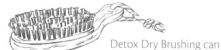

Detox Dry Brushing can be done while you are in the process of practicing Kavala Graha (Detox Oil Swishing). Using a clean, natural-fiber brush while standing in Mountain Pose or seated in Proper Seat, rub the brush over the entire surface of the body (excluding the face). Utilize a steady, firm motion that will create a mild color to the skin, but not so firm as to bruise the skin in any way. Begin brushing from the feet up, working steadily and thoroughly up both legs, back and front, buttocks and belly, up to the heart. Then brush from the hands up the arms, back and front, moving to the chest and back, stroking toward the heart. Detox Dry Brushing will create a soft sheen to the skin by exfoliating the surface as well as help detox the lymphatic system. When finished, rinse the brush with cold water and allow to dry for use again the following day.

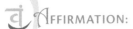 **AFFIRMATION:**

I am clear and filled with good health.

Ingredients needed:

- Mountain Pose
- Organic sea-salt scrub with oil or mild shower soap (optional)
- Singing or humming voice (optional)
- Slow even breaths, inhale equal to exhale
- Gentle Low-Belly Lift (see page 10)

Standing in Mountain Pose, we will stimulate and detox our bodies. A body free of toxins and stress will be stronger, healthier, and younger in appearance. If you want to make this part of your showering routine, use a favorite organic sea-salt scrub with oil or mild soap with the massage. We will stimulate and circulate three areas of the body and with each area explore a bija mantra (seed vibration) to help balance the fluid in each area. Water makes up the majority of our body, and water is very sensitive to vibration, so using sound vibration and light massage will aid your body in flushing and boosting its immune system.

1. Groin—Using the first two finger pads of your dominant hand, lightly massage the side of the lower groin area in a circular motion, moving in the direction of the heart for one minute. If you'd like to add in the sound vibration element, you can either sing the mantra, the sound "lum," or belt out your favorite song. If singing doesn't appeal to you, humming works as well.

2. Under Arms—Moving up to the underarm area, use a gentle, circular stroke with the pads of the first two fingers to massage yourself, which will continue to increase your circulation. Always massage toward the heart. Keep up the vibrational element shifting to the sound of "yum" while massaging for one minute, moving from the forward inner center of the under arm, down through the hollow of the armpit toward the heart, in even, light strokes.

3. Under Jaw—To finish stimulating and detoxing, gently begin a downward stroke toward the heart, beginning right below the jawline at the ear (if adding the vibrational element, shift the sound to "hum" as you move into the this final massage). Again using a soft but steady even pressure, stroke down from jaw through the sides of throat for one minute.

Vibrational Massage or Singing in the Shower

(BIJA MANTRA)

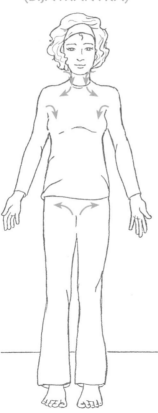

Tree Balance Pose

(VRKSASANA)

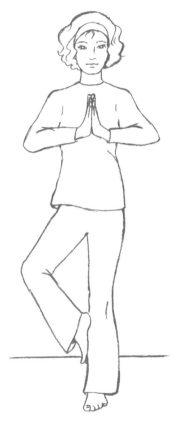

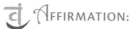

AFFIRMATION:

I am balanced and move with mindfulness.

Ingredients needed:

- Mountain Pose
- Dry, non-slip surface
- One single point of focus
- Slow even breaths, inhale equal to exhale
- Gentle Low-Belly Lift (see page 10)

Now that you are clear, cleansed, and ready to create, we will move into a simple balance to weave our vision of abundance into the rest of the day: our feet being our roots and our hands as an extension of our hearts, intentions moving out into the world steady: balanced, and flexible.

This pose should be done on a non-slip surface, with the body dry and warm.

Stand strong and tall in Mountain Pose with your bare feet hip-width apart, aligned parallel to each other, not turning out or in. Without losing balance, rotate the right leg from deep in the hip socket so the thigh and knee begin to open out to the side. Continue this rotation as you bend the right knee to place the right foot on the inside of your left leg, either below the knee or above the knee but not directly at knee level. Continue to draw the right hip point down, keeping the hip points even, and remain square on the same plane (not elevated or uneven with the other). Breathe evenly to continue to stabilize and draw the chin parallel to the floor holding the gaze on a point at nose level. As you continue to deepen your balance, draw your palms together at your heart center and, if balanced and stable, slowly draw the palms through the midline up toward the ceiling. Once the hands are above the eye line, separate the hands and arms into a V position with fingers spread like rays of the sun to root and raise your intention to the universe.

CHAPTER 3

Fire Up Your Vision of Living

I have the power to create positive change.

Use your thoughts as power.

What is it that you dream of? Do you dream of being more healthy? More courageous? More successful? Today is the day to move closer to your ideal life and dreams. It takes power, discipline, and determination to change negative or unhelpful daily patterns to create the life that we want. It is the small actions that we do throughout the day that will cumulatively bring on large transformations. Our thoughts create our feelings, and our feelings create our actions.

The following yoga practices will shift the status quo to get you off the couch and onto the mat, or in this case onto the living room floor. Yoga Asana(i) (poses or exercises) that activate the core, back, and chest muscles create heat, strength, and stability in the physical body and will also help empower the mind and energize positivity for the rest of the day. Just as with the previous practices, the engine of change is the mind. Repeat the affirmations offered to seed the mind to affirm that you have the strength, power, and energy needed to shift your life into greater abundance. With the mind clear and body feeling strong, you will have increased self-discipline and determination as well as courage to pursue your dreams.

Child's Pose

(BALASANA)

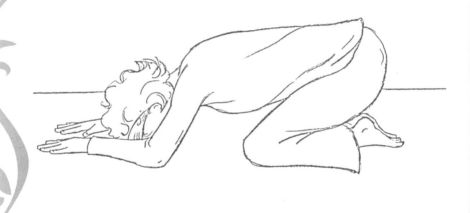

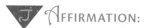

AFFIRMATION:

I am filled with peaceful power.

Ingredients needed:

- Carpet or yoga mat (optional)
- Yoga block or rolled towel (optional)
- Pillow (optional)
- Blanket (optional)
- Slow even breaths, inhale equal to exhale
- Gentle Low-Belly Lift (see page 10)

Starting on the floor kneeling, separate your knees slightly wider than hip width so your belly has room to fully expand when you inhale. Slowly release your torso down toward the floor and rest your forehead on the floor or on your forearms in front of you. (If your forearms are too low to comfortably rest your forehead, a yoga block or a rolled towel can be used instead.) If your forehead is resting on the floor, extend your arms forward, bending the elbows so the hands relax easily on the floor. If there is pressure in the knee joints, place a pillow or rolled towel between the buttocks and the shins, or if there's pressure on the kneecap, add padding such as a blanket underneath the knees. Once comfortable and steady in the pose, continue pressing the forehead on the floor or lifted surface suggested above and breathe five full and complete breaths.

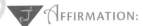

AFFIRMATION:

I am courageous and filled with peaceful power.

Ingredients needed:

- Carpet or yoga mat (optional)
- Slow even breaths, inhale equal to exhale
- Gentle Low-Belly Lift (see page 10)

From Child's Pose, lift up halfway from the floor and align the elbows directly underneath the shoulders. Interlace hands while straightening through the wrists, root forearms into the floor and, with your feet hip-width apart, curl your toes into the floor and lift your hips up and back, away from the floor. Create a small bend in both knees as you continue to press the forearms into the floor and lift from the shoulders to the hips, creating a straight spine. Draw the upper back and shoulder blades in toward the chest as you lengthen the neck and bring the gaze slightly forward of your elbows toward your hands. Utilize full and complete breaths while keeping a firm lift in your core on each exhale. Hold for a minimum of five breaths, increasing duration as is sustainable. To increase stamina and core strength after you have mastered this pose, try a Dolphin Plank Variation by stepping your feet back away from the elbows to bring your body in a straight-line position where the legs are straight and the hips are aligned with the shoulder height while shifting the shoulders forward directly above the elbows.

Dolphin Pose into Child's Pose
(BALASANA)

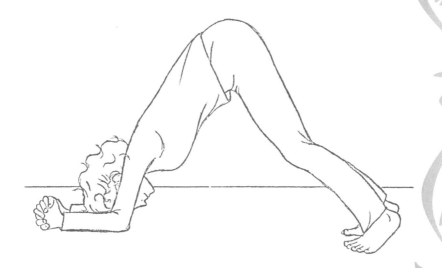

Knees To Chest

(APANASANA)

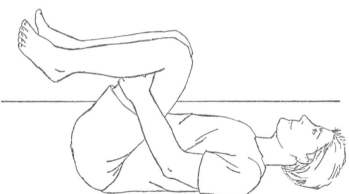

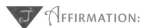

AFFIRMATION:

I am powerful when I let go and go with the flow.

Ingredients needed:

- Carpet or yoga mat (optional)
- Slow even breaths, inhale equal to exhale
- Gentle Low-Belly Lift (see page 10)

Lying on your back, bring your thighs in toward the chest placing your hands behind the thighs. Keeping your head and shoulders rooted to the floor, on the exhale hug your thighs in deeper to press into your chest and belly. Inhale, expand belly and chest and then exhale, pressing thighs into belly. Continue in this dynamic (one movement, one breath) pattern for five breaths total. Lower your feet to the mat and pause for five breaths.

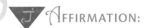

AFFIRMATION:

I am able to shift my challenges to opportunities.

Ingredients needed:

- Carpet or yoga mat (optional)
- Yoga block (optional)
- Slow even breaths, inhale equal to exhale
- Gentle Low-Belly Lift (see page 10)

Lying on your back, place your hands or forearms under the buttocks, palms facing down, to support the low back. Root the back of the shoulders and the back of the head (gently) to the floor and keep them rooted throughout the duration of this exercise. Draw the knees in toward the chest, stopping with your knees directly over the hip points. Activate the core to support the legs in this position and hug the thighs toward the midline so they remain parallel and hip-width apart. If you have a yoga block, place the block thin-wise three inches down from the groin and three inches up from the knees and squeeze the block to stabilize the core and low back. This is a great option for those with low-back issues. If using a yoga block, continue with the block in place throughout the exercise. Begin to straighten the legs and bring the feet toward the ceiling, making sure to straighten only as far as there is no strain or pulling sensation on the low back. If you are not using a yoga block, slowly begin to lower just the right leg to where it sustainably hovers over the floor; this hover can be a few feet or a few inches. The key here is steady work but no strain in the low back or neck. Keeping the shoulders and back of the head on the mat, begin to slowly alternate lifting and lowering each leg one breath at a time. Move only on the exhales and pause on the inhales to expand the neck and fuel the practice. If utilizing a block or if you have low-back issues, keep the legs together; and if there is a feeling of strain in the low back, do the exercise with bent knees the entire time. Begin with five to ten full cycles and increase as is sustainable. Hug the thighs in toward the chest in Knees to Chest Pose (see page 42) to finish releasing the low back and core for five breaths to complete.

Alternative Leg Lifts
(EKA PADA URDHVA PRASARITA PADOTTANASANA)

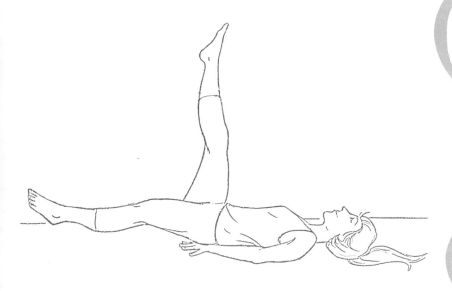

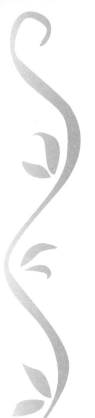

Yogi Bicycles
(EKA PADA NAVASANA)

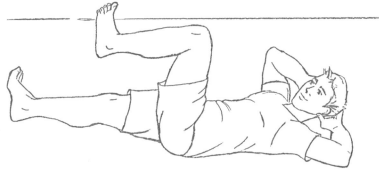

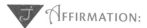

AFFIRMATION:

I am strong and intentional.

Ingredients needed:

- Carpet or yoga mat (optional)
- Slow even breaths, inhale equal to exhale
- Gentle Low-Belly Lift (see page 10)

Lying on your back, bring your knees in toward your chest. Bring your fingertips to the back of both sides of your head to support its weight. Open the chest by broadening the collarbones and move the bent elbows out to the sides. Keep the elbows out to the side and a fist's distance between the chin and collarbones throughout the duration of this series. Use the core muscles (not the neck) to lift the shoulders two inches off the floor, then extend the left leg straight, hovering a few inches over the floor while you twist from the navel and bring the left shoulder closer to the right knee while you slowly exhale. Next, slowly inhale and switch to extending the right leg straight, hovering over the floor, and then exhale as you draw the left knee in toward the core and the right shoulder toward the knee. Continue to alternate the position of the legs and shoulders while you continue to inhale and exhale. Remember, this is a movement from your body's core, not from the shoulders or neck. Begin with five to ten full cycles and increase amount as is sustainable. If you have any low-back issues or discomfort, keep a bend in both knees and lightly rest the toes on the floor during each cycle. End this exercise by hugging the thighs into the belly in Knees to Chest Pose (see page 42) and then rolling to your left side in fetal position to rest for ten breaths before getting up.

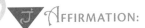

AFFIRMATION:

I burn away any fear and open to love.

Ingredients needed:

- Carpet or yoga mat (optional)
- Yoga block (optional)
- Yoga strap or hand towel (optional)
- Slow even breaths, inhale equal to exhale
- Gentle Low-Belly Lift (see page 10)

Lying on the belly with the forehead down, straighten the legs and set the feet hip-width apart. Point the toes and root the tops of the feet to the floor. Firm the thigh muscles to keep the feet rooted throughout this exercise. Inhale and lengthen through the torso, bringing the sternum toward the crown of the head and then stretch the arms back behind you as if you were reaching toward your feet. Lift the hands off the floor and, if possible, clasp the thumbs together behind you above the buttocks. If you cannot easily clasp your thumbs together while straightening the elbows, hold either a yoga strap or hand towel between your hands, shoulder-width apart. Activate the thighs and root the tops of the feet into the floor. While inhaling, begin to lift the chest, shoulders, and head a few inches off the mat and then as you exhale, slowly lower back down. Continue lifting on the inhale and slowly lowering back down as you exhale. Be sure to use the muscles in the legs and upper back to lift in this pose, not the head and neck. Do three sets of five dynamic lifts on the breath before moving on to the next exercise. Once complete, release the arms and turn one ear to the floor. Rest for five to ten breaths, turn your head back to center, and then turn your head so the opposite ear rests on the floor to release the neck on the other side as well.

Locust Pose with Hand Clasp

(SALABHASANA C CLASP)

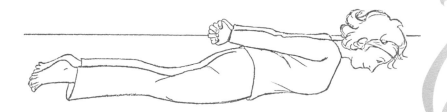

Bridge Pose
(SETU BANDHA)

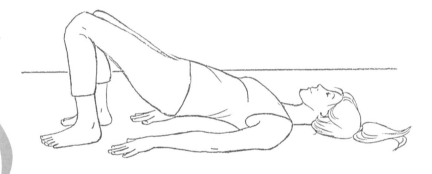

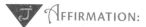

Affirmation:

I am ready to live my ideal life.

Ingredients needed:

- Carpet or yoga mat (optional)
- Yoga block (optional)
- Slow even breaths, inhale equal to exhale
- Gentle Low-Belly Lift (see page 10)

Begin by lying on your back with your knees bent and your feet parallel and hip-width apart, knees stacked directly over your heels. Root the back of the shoulders and back of the head (gently) down to the floor where they will remain for the duration of this exercise. Straighten the arms and place the palms face down directly beside the hips and begin to root feet, hands, shoulders to the floor. While inhaling, slowly lift the hips toward the ceiling, stopping at about seventy-five percent capacity, while continuing to keep the thighs hip-width apart. Next, exhale and slowly lower the hips back down to the floor. Continue lifting upon inhale and lowering upon exhale in a dynamic one movement, one breath. On the fifth cycle, stop while the hips are up, aligning thighs hip-width apart, and hold while breathing for five breaths; then slowly lower back to the floor. Do three sets of five lifts and holds before moving on to the next exercise. Once completed, lower the hips down to the floor and separate the feet to twice as wide as your hip width, releasing the knees slowly to the midline to touch. Breathe in that position for five to ten breaths before moving.

Knees to Chest Pose
(APANASANA)

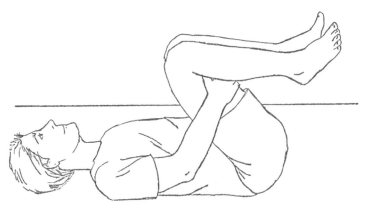

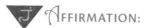

I will take my courage and power into the rest of my day.

Ingredients needed:

- Carpet or yoga mat (optional)
- Slow even breaths, inhale equal to exhale
- Gentle Low-Belly Lift (see page 10)

Lying on your back with shoulders and head gently rooted to the floor, hug the thighs into the belly while holding the back of the thighs with your hands. Inhale and widen through the collarbones and then exhale and draw the thighs into the belly until they're pressing the abdomen. Create a gentle, slow rhythm on the inhale and exhale, repeating for five cycles and then roll to the left side in a fetal position. As you get back up, consciously focus on living out the rest of your day connected to your envisioned goal or purpose.

CHAPTER 4

Moving Out and About

I love and forgive myself.

True strength is from

When we feel good, we do good. And now that we have cultivated a strong, positive outlook, a light, detoxed body, and a stable core, we are fired up to get strong. True strength is not only from power but also from relaxed flexibility. A balance of abhyasa (consistent practice, "just keep going," which makes us strong) and vairagya (open-hearted acceptance and forgiveness, "oh well!" which makes us joyful) will allow compassion to flow and healing energy to move through all aspects of our body and life. In plain language, just get out there and do your yoga. Don't overthink it or stress about it, allow it to be light and fun.

Doing yoga anywhere and everywhere holds such delight for me personally. Take this joyful practice, that will tone your legs and heart, with you to the gym, work, on your travels, or like me to the yard with kids, without shoes, and pretty much everywhere else you go.

power and flexibility.

Chair Pose

(UTKATASANA)

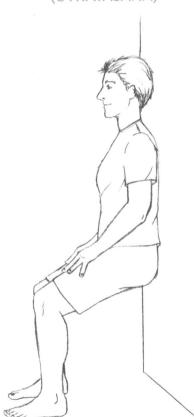

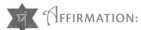 **AFFIRMATION:**

I am most effective when I am simultaneously strong and relaxed.

Ingredients needed:

- Wall (optional)
- Yoga block (optional)
- Slow even breaths, inhale equal to exhale
- Gentle Low-Belly Lift (see page 10)

Align your feet hip-width apart and parallel to each other, not turned out or in. Bend the knees and shift your body weight toward the heels as you move your hips toward the floor as if attempting to sit onto a chair. Keep the knees straight ahead in line with the second toe of each foot and, as you sit, lengthen down through the tailbone as you firm the belly and lift up through the sternum creating a straight spine. Place your hands on the hip points for balance and lift your chin parallel to the floor creating a focus straight ahead. Lower to where you are balanced and stable, yet building strength in sustainable challenge. Breathe full and complete breaths, holding this relaxed focus ten to fifteen breaths and then slowly, pressing into the floor, rise from belly to crown of head to stand. Stand in Mountain Pose for five steady breaths alternating with stillness. Do three cycles of Chair into Mountain Pose, slowly increasing strength and capacity to hold longer durations as you practice. If you have any low-back or knee issues, use a wall to support yourself while you sit, squaring the pelvis to the wall and aligning the heels directly underneath the knees to help stabilize the hips and support the low-back and knee joints.

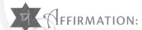

AFFIRMATION:

I am right where I need to be.

Ingredients needed:

- Slow even breaths, inhale equal to exhale
- Gentle Low-Belly Lift (see page 10)

Standing in Mountain Pose, open your arms straight out to the sides in T position. Step your feet out as wide as your fingertips. Come up on the toes of the right foot and rotate the leg from deep in the hip socket to rotate the right thigh, then knee, and foot to the side so the right heel is in alignment with the arch of the left foot. Align the right knee with the second toe of the right foot while bending the right knee to stop directly over the ankle of the right foot. If the knee passes the ankle, step your feet a little wider apart so you have the correct, sustainable-yet-strengthening pose. If you feel unstable, bring your hands to the hip points and focus on slowing the breath. Breathe full, complete breaths as you remain in the posture, lifting the front right hip point to balance the pelvis and lengthen the tailbone down toward the floor as you firm the belly and lift the sternum up to lengthen the spine. Bring your gaze toward the right hand and turn the palms to face up as you repeat your positive intention and affirmation for this pose. Breathe ten to fifteen slow cycles, and then slowly root the right heel and rise up through the rest of the body to come to straight legs. Step feet back together in Mountain Pose and breathe in stillness for five breaths. Follow the above directions, switching left leg for right. Always do both sides of any asymmetric exercise such as this to cultivate even balance and strength on both sides. Finish by stepping the feet together in Mountain Pose and breathing in stillness for five breaths.

Warrior 2 Pose

(VIRADBHADRASANA 2)

Revolving Chair Pose

(PARIVRTTA UTKATASANA)

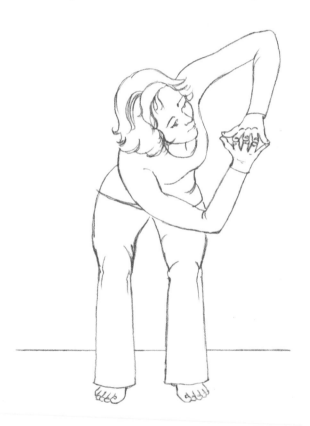

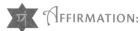

AFFIRMATION:

I accept what is and trust the timing.

Ingredients needed:

- Wall (optional)
- Yoga block (optional)
- Slow even breaths, inhale equal to exhale
- Gentle Low-Belly Lift (see page 10)

Begin in Chair Pose and then draw your palms to touch at the center of the chest. Activate the thighs and firm the belly to ensure that the hips do not twist but remain square and stable. Inhale to lengthen through the spine and, as you exhale from the core, begin to twist and then place the right elbow on the outside of the left thigh. Do not initiate the twist from the hips and low back. Make sure it is initiating from the belly and moving in the upper back directly behind the heart center under the rib cage. Continue to breathe full and complete breaths, inhaling to lengthen the spine and exhaling to gently twist from belly into upper back for five to seven cycles. Slowly release and fold into an easy forward fold for five slow breaths and then slowly, with control, return to Chair Pose. Follow the previous instructions but now twist to bring the left elbow to the outside of the right thigh, breathing for five to seven breaths and then once again folding into an easy forward fold. When this full practice is complete, slowly and deliberately inhale to rise with a flat back and soft knees to stand in Mountain Pose for five steady breaths and stillness before moving on to the next practice. As with Chair Pose, consider if you have any low-back or knee issues and utilize a wall to sit in Chair position before twisting, which will help stabilize the hips and support the low-back and knee joints.

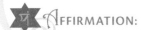

AFFIRMATION:

I am filled with compassion and purged of fear.

Ingredients needed:

- Slow even breaths, inhale equal to exhale
- Gentle Low-Belly Lift (see page 10)

From Mountain Pose, bring your hands to the hip points for balance and firm the core muscles. On an exhale step the left foot about one leg length back behind you in lunge position. Firm the right outer hip muscles to align the front right knee directly over the ankle and in line with the second toe of the right foot. Bring the back left hip forward to square the hips evenly. If you feel unstable, consider stepping the back foot a few inches forward for a shorter stance. Soften the back left knee slightly toward the floor and, as you lengthen the tailbone down, firm the belly and lift the sternum, drawing the spine straight and lifting the chest and head. Lift the chin parallel to the floor, holding your gaze at nose height. Inhale and continue to lift the chest and lengthen the spine exhale firming the thighs toward the midline and the belly in to stabilize. Breathe five to ten full and complete cycles of breath, then with hands on the hip points, firm the belly and shift the back left foot up to meet the right, continuing to have the feet hip-width apart and parallel to each other, and step back into Mountain Pose. Repeat the pose, alternating to the other side: left foot forward, right foot back. To finish, gently step back into Mountain Pose for five steady breaths and stillness before moving on to the next practice.

Crescent Lunge

(ANJANEYASANA)

Standing Back-bend

(ANUVITTASANA)

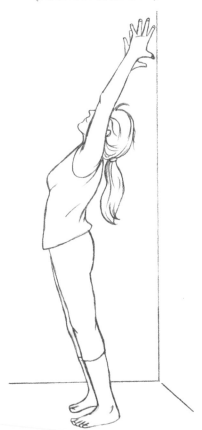

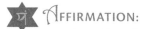

Affirmation:

I am able to give and receive love.

Ingredients needed:

- Wall (optional)
- Yoga block (optional)
- Slow even breaths, inhale equal to exhale
- Gentle Low-Belly Lift (see page 10)

Standing in Mountain Pose, align body an arm's length from a wall, then turn with your back toward the wall, root your feet evenly into the floor, and firm the thighs and belly to stabilize the low back. Continue to root as you inhale and stretch the arms forward and up on either side of the head, straightening the arms and opening the palms so they face each other. If you have any pain in your low back or tightness in your neck, widen the arms to a V and stop there, keeping the arms overhead or slightly forward, and breathe. If you feel stable with no strain, continue to work the legs and belly to stabilize while you inhale deeper and extend your arms and thumbs back to lightly touch the wall behind you in a standing back-bend. Exhale, firming the thighs and belly strongly as you inhale to lengthen spine, lifting up and back. Breathe five to seven full and complete breaths and then slowly firm the belly and exhale the arms back down to your sides. Stand in Mountain Pose in stillness to reset before doing two more cycles of this Standing Back-bend series. On the final Mountain Pose, hold for five to ten breaths, feeling the effects of the practice.

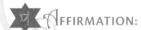

AFFIRMATION:

I am full of vitality and joy.

Ingredients needed:

- Chair or wall (optional)
- Slow even breaths, inhale equal to exhale
- Gentle Low-Belly Lift (see page 10)

Begin in Chair Pose. With weight evenly rooted on the left side of the body, firm the core and rotate the right thighbone in the hip socket as you did previously in the Warrior 2 Pose. Cross the right shin or ankle over the left thigh. Draw the right side of the hip down, as it may have lifted in this process, to stabilize the low back while keeping the balance and position of Chair Pose. Flex the right foot, straightening the ankle. Firm the belly and lift the sternum to lengthen the spine. Lift the chin parallel to the floor and focus your gaze and intention at nose height. Hold for ten to fifteen breaths before uncrossing the top leg and standing in Mountain Pose for five breaths of stillness. Do the other side as previously instructed. To finish the pose, stand in Mountain Pose for five steady breaths and stillness before moving on to the next practice or the next adventure of the day.

Cross-Legged Chair Pose

(UTKATSANA SUCIRANDHRASANA)

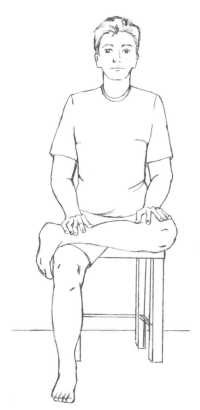

CHAPTER 5

Sharing Space for Truth and Grace

I speak my truth from a state of love and gratitude.

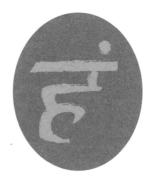

Create silence
and listen.

In my life, learning how to speak my truth has been one of my challenges. Even more challenging has been knowing when to keep my mouth shut and listen. Each of us has a gift and contribution to the world. Our truth is as unique as an individual snowflake and originates from our universal essence of pure love, grace, and gratitude. As I have said before, what we think, we become, and when we feel good, we do good. When we are intentionally creating and healing our body and life, then we have greater clarity in our sharing in the world. When we share our highest selves with the world, it feels good and can be a weight off our heart and shoulders. We have been building this clarity and power through our previous chapters' practices. The sharing of our truth can be big or as sweetly simple as our offering of gratitude to others or saying "grace" at mealtime.

Sometimes the greatest space of communication is sharing ourselves, while other times we allow space for listening. The power to be able to be still, quiet, and listen is profound. When in doubt of what to express, allow for silence and turn to compassionate listening. When about to speak, pause and place it through the filter of: Is it true? Is it kind with the intention of the greater good? Is it imperative? If the answer to any of these is "No," then pause, create silence, and listen. In this balance of sharing and listening, we create a profound exchange with each other.

These practices will enhance your ability to authentically communicate as well as listen effectively. They can be done at any point during the day and in most any location, even in the car. They are especially useful in preparing for important communications, whether at home, work, or simply during connection at mealtime. The Neck Rolls, Lion's Breath, and Vocalizing will also release neck and jaw tightness, which is great for relieving tension headaches and neck aches.

Neck Rolls (3 Variations)
(GRIVA VINYASA)

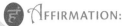

AFFIRMATION:

I speak with kindness even when it is difficult.

Ingredients needed:

- Proper Seat or Mountain Pose
- Slow even breaths, inhale equal to exhale
- Gentle Low-Belly Lift (see page 10)

Begin in either Chair Pose or Mountain Pose, with palms pressed into the low belly for core support. Place your tongue behind your bottom teeth and inhale through the nose. Then, as you exhale, vigorously press the tongue to the back of the teeth to force the root of the tongue up and out toward the front of the mouth. As the tongue pushes forward, create a "hah" without vibration to begin. Next, once comfortable with that action and breath working together, add a sighing type of vibration with your vocal chords on the exhale. Finally, force the tongue out of the body and "roar" like a lion full of passion, purpose, and peaceful power. After the initial practice rounds, do three additional rounds. Although there is sound coming from the vocal chords, this is still to be a fairly gentle massage, not jarring or harming to the throat. If you have any hoarseness or soreness as a result of this exercise, you are pushing too hard and should be gentler next time.

Lion's Breath
(SIMHASANA)

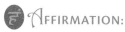 **AFFIRMATION:**

I manifest my highest good and the good of others.

Ingredients needed:

- Proper Seat or Mountain Pose
- Slow even breaths, inhale equal to exhale
- Gentle Low-Belly Lift (see page 10)

Begin in either Proper Seat or Mountain Pose, with palms pressed into the low belly for core support. Stabilize the body into its foundation and lengthen the spine by lifting and opening the chest.

1. With the head aligned straight ahead, chin parallel to the floor, inhale and gently turn the face toward the right side of the body. On the exhale, slowly return back to center. Repeat the other direction, on the inhale, gently turn the face toward the left side of the body, and on the exhale slowly return to center. Repeat these movements and breaths to complete five full cycles (right and left).

2. From center position with the head aligned straight ahead, chin parallel to the floor, inhale and gently draw the right ear toward the right shoulder. On the exhale, slowly return the head up right to center. Repeat the other direction on the inhale, gently draw the left ear towards the left shoulder and on the exhale slowly return back to center. Repeat these movements and breaths to complete five full cycles.

3. From center position with the head aligned straight ahead, chin parallel to the floor, inhale and gently draw the nose toward the right shoulder, creating a diagonal stretch on the exhale, slowly return the head up right to center. Repeat the other direction by inhaling as you gently draw the nose toward the left shoulder and exhaling as you slowly return back to center. Repeat these movements and breaths to complete five full cycles.

To finish, return your head back to center with the chin parallel to the floor and do five full and complete breaths and stillness before moving on to the next practice.

Mouth Lip Rolls

(MUKHAM ADHARA VINYASA)

 AFFIRMATION: *I am an instrument of truth, love, and abundance.*

Ingredients needed:

- Proper Seat or Mountain Pose
- Slow even breaths, inhale equal to exhale
- Gentle Low-Belly Lift (see page 10)

Begin in either Chair Pose or Mountain Pose, with palms pressed into the low belly for core support.

Lemon Sandwich Mouth Chews—Open the mouth as if you were to bite into an oversize sandwich and then purse lips like you are tasting something extremely sour.

Repeat for five to ten chews.

Blowing through the lips—Keeping lips lightly touching, blow air through them as if you were to blow bubbles. Relax the face so the lips bounce on each other creating vibration and release. Once comfortable with this process, add a sigh-like breath behind the blowing, moving high and low on the octave in your voice.

Practice ten to thirty blows

"Meow" like you mean it—Focusing the meow up behind the nose and vibrating the soft palate. If the nose begins to tickle, you are doing it just right. If you begin to giggle, you receive extra credit.

Practice ten to thirty meows.

Cutting and Shaping your communication—Work through the consonants below one time very slowly and deliberately and then three times a little faster. Be sure to make the sounds crisply and clearly. Finally, repeat them ten times, still crisply and clearly. If the sounds become blurred or muddy, begin the process over again.

P. T. K. PTKPTKPTK. PTKPTKPTKPTKPTKPTKPTKPTKPTKPTKPTK.
B. D. G. BDGBDGBDG. BDGBDGBDGBDGBDGBDGBDGBDGBDGBDGBDG
K.G.nG. KGnGKGnGKGnG. KGnGKGnGKGnGKGnGKGnGKGnGKGnGKGKG
S.Sh.Zz S.Sh.Zz S.Sh.Zz   S.Sh.Zz S.Sh.Zz S.Sh.Zz S.Sh.Zz S.Sh.Zz S.Sh.Zz

HOOM HUM BRAHM HUM—Sing or vibrate through the warming and opening sounds of HOOM HUM BRAHM HUM. May you be able to speak and listen, honoring your truth, kindness, and wisdom.

Repeat ten to thirty vibrations

Deep Listening Meditation
(ANTAR MOUNA)

 AFFIRMATION: *I listen with an open heart.*

Ingredients needed:

- Proper Seat, lying down, or Mountain Pose
- Slow even breaths, inhale equal to exhale
- Stillness
- Gentle Low-Belly Lift (see page 10)

In Proper Seat, lying down, or Mountain Pose, we will begin creating an awareness of the conscious workings of the mind and thoughts. When we become conscious of our thoughts and can transform them, then we direct our mind to freedom. Begin with your eyes closed, slow down your breathing, and consciously create slow, even breaths with the inhale equal to the exhale.

Become aware of sensations in the body, starting at the bottoms of your feet. Slowly begin to guide your awareness from your feet to your knees, into the hip sockets, to the center of the belly at the navel, into the center of the chest, and then to your elbows and hands. Return to the chest center and slowly continue the sensation, tracking into the center of the throat and then residing in between the eyebrows. While you progress tracking, become a passive observer of your sensations as well as your thoughts. Untangle yourself from the cycle of thoughts and reactions. This Deep Listening Meditation will create freedom and clarity, allowing you to cultivate the thoughts of love and gratitude and create a powerful shift in your next actions. It can be done at any point within your day, although I recommend choosing to add it before busy transitions or any activity that may have more challenge or stress involved. I often utilize this meditation either before I turn the ignition to drive my car or after I have turned my ignition off and am about to move into a meeting or more-involved task.

Counting Blessings
(KRITAGYATA)

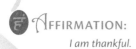

AFFIRMATION:
I am thankful.

Ingredients needed:

- Proper Seat or Mountain Pose
- Stillness
- Slow even breaths, inhale equal to exhale
- Gentle Low-Belly Lift (see page 10)

Counting Blessings can be practiced separately or in conjunction with the Deep Listening Meditation (see page 76). From wherever you are in your daily routine, pause and practice slow, even breaths. In a place of stillness, begin to count your blessing by writing them down or simply saying them out loud or silently to yourself. Count the most basic blessings that you may disregard or take for granted, such as sleeping in a warm bed or drinking clean water, and build to what may be considered the most significant gratitudes such as the loves in your life or grand abundances. When you have completed counting your blessings, hold the space of breathing and stillness for five breaths before moving on to the next task in your day.

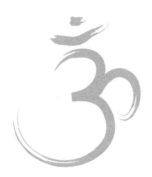

CHAPTER 6

Cultivating Rest and Peace

I trust my intuition.

Set up a ritual for relaxation.

The ability to rest and relax is the most powerful practice of all. Moving from a stress response (go go go!) to a restore response (ahhhh!) will benefit your mind, body, and life. When we relax the mind and body, we also improve mental clarity, our ability to focus, and our creativity; as well, we balance our emotions and create greater enjoyment of life.

In this final chapter, we will set up a ritual for relaxation, connection, and healing to open our innate wisdom and intuition. When we are free of stress and immersed in restful, abundant peace, we are able to truly feel our connectedness to the divine, the world, and each other.

In the previous chapters, we have explored the ingredients for a heart-connected and abundant life. This exploration prepared us for the full Relaxation Recipe, which is when we simultaneously repeat an awareness, movement, or practice (in the following exercises, it will be repetition of breath awareness and or affirmation) while remaining in a state of passive disregard. This is a deep version of Abhyasa and Vairagya, consistently practicing (just keep going!) while being unconcerned with how it will turn out (oh well!).

When we grip anything too tightly, we will stifle it, but if we hold it easily, compassionately open to possibility, it can lift off and fly. Daily, consistent practice (just keep going!) while being unconcerned with how it will turn out (oh well!) is the magic recipe that will affect all aspects of life and be especially helpful when utilizing the tools of relaxation and sleep preparation.

After you have prepared for bed, practice the Relaxation Recipe with the following exercises of unwinding; this coupling will lead you into peace and eventually into healing sleep.

Child's Pose and Knees to Chest

(BALASANA) AND (APANASANA)

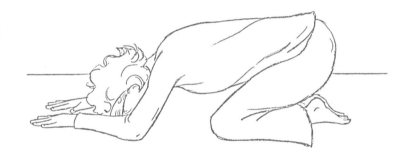

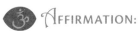

AFFIRMATION:

I accept what is and trust the timing.

Ingredients needed:

- Floor, mattress or yoga mat (optional)

- Slow even breaths, inhale equal to exhale

- Gentle Low-Belly Lift (see page 10)

Begin in Child's Pose (see page 38) taking at least ten slow breaths to begin to quiet. Once you feel grounded and quiet, slowly transition on to your back. Keeping your head and shoulders rooted to the floor, hug your thighs in towards your chest for Knee to Chest Pose (see page 52).

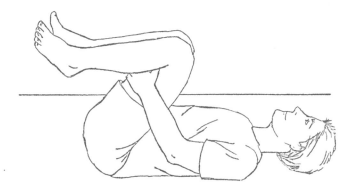

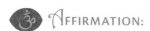

AFFIRMATION:

I am free and release anything not in my power.

Ingredients needed:

- Floor, mattress, or yoga mat (optional)
- Slow even breaths, inhale equal to exhale
- Inhale, lengthen spine, exhale, twist
- Gentle Low-Belly Lift (see page 10)

Lying on your back with Knees to Chest (see page 42), firm the core muscles and, on a slow three count, draw the thighs over to the left of the body to eventually rest on the floor. Continue to firm the belly and draw the thighs toward the chest to where you feel a sustainable wringing-out pressure on the abdomen. Inhale and lengthen through the right side of the waist, lengthening the sternum away from the hips and then exhale deeper and draw the right shoulder down toward the floor to expand the chest and increasingly open the breath and collarbones. With full and complete breaths, inhale and lengthen through the spine. On each exhale, firm the belly and deepen the twist, wringing out toxins from the deep belly and spine. When complete on this side, hug the thighs together, engage the core muscles, and slowly on a three count, return to your back, with head and shoulders on the floor and thighs into belly. Stay for a few breaths and then, on the next exhale, firm the belly and on a three count, slowly lower the thighs in the opposite direction, and twist once again following the instructions utilized for side one. Return to thighs into chest for a gentle hugging squeeze and then roll on to your left side in fetal position with the left forearm supporting the head before transitioning to the next practice.

Simple Twist
(JATHARA PARIVARTINASANA)

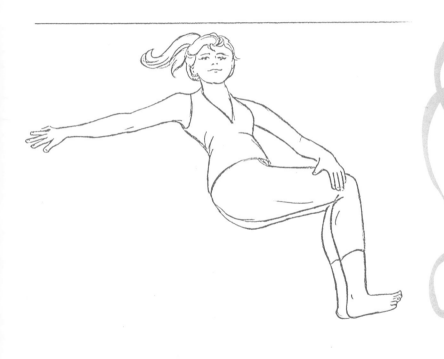

Legs Up the Wall

(VIPARITA KARANI)

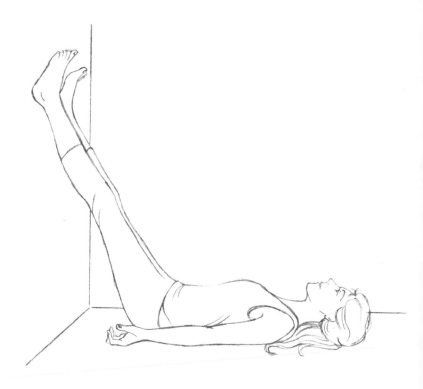

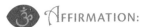

AFFIRMATION:

I am supported by universal love.

Ingredients needed:

- Floor, mattress or yoga mat (optional)
- Slow even breaths, inhale equal to exhale
- Gentle Low-Belly Lift (see page 10)

In a fetal position, approximately six to eight inches away from a wall or headboard of a bed, firm the belly to slowly transition onto the back, lifting the right leg to extend up the wall followed by the left leg until both legs are straight up the wall. Bring the hips to evenly square up to the wall but not against the wall, still six to eight inches away so there is room for the tailbone to release and not be curled up. If the tailbone is curled toward the wall or there is any strain in the low back, bend the knees to plant the feet on the wall and gently shift the body another three to five inches away from the wall or until the strain is released. Create symmetry on both the right and left sides of the body including the arms and hands. Place the hands palms-down on the low belly between the navel and pubis or open toward the ceiling out to the sides of the body. Close the eyes and breathe thirty cycles of full and complete breaths. Once completed, bend the knees into the chest and, with a firm belly, slowly hug the thighs in and release once again into a fetal position on the left side. Support the head with the bottom arm and breathe five slow breaths before mindfully using the top hand to come upright for the next posture.

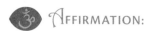

ॐ AFFIRMATION:

I am held and a bridge to the infinite.

Ingredients needed:

- Floor, mattress, or yoga mat (optional)
- Yoga block, bolster, or large rolled towel
- Slow even breaths, inhale equal to exhale
- Gentle Low-Belly Lift (see page 10)

This pose will release the low back by opening the hips and prepare you for relaxation and sleep. Begin by sitting cross-legged with your sitting bones on a firm pillow, rolled towel, or yoga block. Anchor the hips evenly with the knees sloping down to create a stable, low triangle. Lift the chest and sternum to lengthen the spine. Align the elbows underneath the shoulder joints. Align the head and shoulders directly over the hips, keeping a straight spine, and close the eyes.

To align the mind, bring your attention to the tip of your nose and breathe a full and complete breath. Deeply inhale from the tip of your nose through both nostrils, resting your awareness in between your eyebrows and then evenly exhale back down through both nostrils, once again resting your awareness at the tip of the nose. Continue with the breath awareness for one to two minutes or until a sensation of deep calm or sleepiness occurs.

Once finished, briefly open your eyes to stabilize and switch which leg is crossed on top of the other. Sit upright and do a second round of the above guided breath. When both sides of the breath cycle are complete, begin to gently massage from the hip socket of the upper leg down through the thigh, calf, and foot. End by squeezing each of the toes and then do the same from the hip socket of the other leg, working through the entire leg and foot before coming back upright and shifting to recline on the back for the final quieting exercise.

Easy Seat Quieting Meditation and Massage

(NADI SHODHANA VARIATION SUKHASANA)

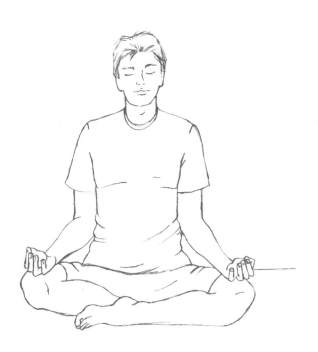

Corpse Pose with Focus of Awareness Healing

(SAVASANA)

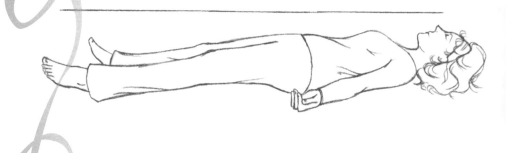

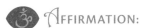 ᚱFFIRMATION:

I am a conduit of unbound love and healing.

Ingredients needed:

- Floor, mattress, or yoga mat (optional)
- Yoga block, bolster, or large rolled towel
- Slow even breaths, inhale equal to exhale

Lying on your back with straight legs slightly separated and open thighs, straighten your arms and place them with the palms up, five inches away from the torso, in a symmetrical, reclined shape. If you feel discomfort in your low back, add a yoga bolster or large, rolled bath towel underneath the knees. Close your eyes and allow your face and eyeballs to soften. Begin to extend the exhale slightly longer than the inhale and begin to create a quiet heaviness in the body. If you fall asleep here, wonderful! Happy resting! If you're still awake, move on to the Forty-one Focus of Awareness Meditation to close your powerful, intentional day of practice.

Forty-one Focus
of Awareness Meditation

While remaining in the open, quiet state of Corpse Pose, cycle through the following forty-one visualizing and breathing practices. Do three cycles of full and complete breaths for each and consider adding the affirmation of love and healing on each awareness.

Inhale, focusing on the center of the eyebrows, then slowly exhale.
Inhale, focusing on the center of the throat, then slowly exhale.
Inhale, focusing on the center of the chest, then slowly exhale.
Inhale, focusing on the center of the right shoulder joint, then slowly exhale.
Inhale, focusing on the center of the right elbow joint, then slowly exhale.
Inhale, focusing on the center of the right wrist joint, then slowly exhale.
Inhale, focusing on the center of the right palm through all fingers, then slowly exhale.
Inhale, focusing on the center of the right wrist joint , then slowly exhale.
Inhale, focusing on the center of the right elbow joint, then slowly exhale.
Inhale, focusing on the center of the right shoulder joint, then slowly exhale.
Inhale, focusing on the center of the chest, then slowly exhale.
Inhale, focusing on the center of the left shoulder joint, then slowly exhale.
Inhale, focusing on the center of the left elbow joint, then slowly exhale.
Inhale, focusing on the center of the left wrist joint, then slowly exhale.
Inhale, focusing on the center of the left palm through all fingers, then slowly exhale.
Inhale, focusing on the center of the left wrist joint, then slowly exhale.
Inhale, focusing on the center of the left elbow joint, then slowly exhale.
Inhale, focusing on the center of the left shoulder joint, then slowly exhale.
Inhale, focusing on the center of the chest, then slowly exhale.
Inhale, focusing on the center of the navel, then slowly exhale.
Inhale, focusing on the center of the lower-belly pelvic bowl, then slowly exhale

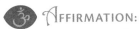

AFFIRMATION:

I am a conduit of unbound love and healing.

Inhale, focusing on the center of the right hip joint, then slowly exhale.
Inhale, focusing on the center of the right knee joint, then slowly exhale.
Inhale, focusing on the center of the right ankle joint, then slowly exhale.
Inhale, focusing on the center of the right sole of the foot through the toes, then slowly exhale.
Inhale, focusing on the center of the right ankle joint, then slowly exhale.
Inhale, focusing on the center of the right knee joint, then slowly exhale.
Inhale, focusing on the center of the right hip joint, then slowly exhale.
Inhale, focusing on the center of the lower-belly pelvic bowl, then slowly exhale.
Inhale, focusing on the center of the left hip joint, then slowly exhale.
Inhale, focusing on the center of the left knee joint, then slowly exhale.
Inhale, focusing on the center of the left ankle joint, then slowly exhale.
Inhale, focusing on the center of the left sole of the foot through the toes, then slowly exhale.
Inhale, focusing on the center of the left ankle joint, then slowly exhale.
Inhale, focusing on the center of the left knee joint, then slowly exhale.
Inhale, focusing on the center of the left hip joint, then slowly exhale.
Inhale, focusing on the center of the pelvic bowl, then slowly exhale.
Inhale, focusing on the center of the navel, then slowly exhale.
Inhale, focusing on the center of the chest, then slowly exhale.
Inhale, focusing on the center of the throat, then slowly exhale.
Inhale, focusing on the center of the eyebrows (intuition command center),
   then slowly exhale for ten breaths.

Glossary

Abhyasa: a consistent, balanced practice or effort (just keep going!)

Adho Mukha Svanasana (modified): an asana, modified Downward-Facing Dog or Puppy Dog Pose

Affirmation: a positive phrase of encouragement; resetting negative thinking into positive

Ama: toxins

Anjaneyasana: an asana; Crescent Lunge Pose

Antar Mouna: a meditation practice; creating silence for interior or deep listening

Anuvittasana: an asana; Standing Back-Bending Pose

Apanasana: an asana; Knees to Chest Pose

Asana: a posture, position, or pose for meditation or yoga; asani for multiple postures

Balasana: an asana; Child's Pose

Bija: seed or source; bija mantra sacred sound or vibration that correlates with emotional nerve plexus in body or Chakra; lum, yum, hum

Chakra: a wheel of life force that correlates with the nerve plexus in the body

Dynamic Movement: movement synch with breath; one movement, one breath

Eka Pada Navasana: an asana; Yogi Bicycle Pose

Eka Pada Urdhva Prasarita Padottanasana: an asana; Alternative Leg Lifts

Griva Vinyasa: an asana series; Neck Movements or Rolls on the Breath

Ihiva Kriya: Tongue Scraping cleansing practice

Jathara Parivartinasana: an asana; simple supine twist or passive belly churning

Kavala Graha Kriya: Detox Oil Swishing cleansing technique

Kritagyata: gratitude

Kriya: cleansing practice or technique

Malasana (modified): an asana; Standing High Squat or Goddess Pose

Mantra: a sacred sound, word, phrase or affirmation

Mouna: silence as a spiritual practice to listen

Mukham Adhara Vinyasa: an asani series; face, mouth, lip movements on breath

Mulabhanda; a pelvic floor, Gentle Low-Belly Lift or lock; similar to a "kegel"

Nadi Shodhana: a pranayama; alternating nostril balancing

Namaste: an expression loosely translated as "the light and love in me recognizes and bows to that in you"

Parivrtta Tadasana: an asana; upright standing twist in Mountain Pose

Parivrtta Utkatasana: an asana; twisted Chair Pose

Prana: life force

Pranayama: breathing exercise or technique that directs life force

Prasarita Padottanasana A (modified): an asana; Soft-Kneed Wide Leg Forward Fold modified with bent or soft knees

Salabhasana C Clasp: an asana; Locust Pose with hands clasped behind the back

Savasana: an asana; Corpse Pose

Setu Bandha: an asana; Bridge Pose

Simhasana: an asana/pranayama: Lion's Breath Pose

Sukhasana; an asana; cross-legged "comfortable" seat

Tadasana: an asana; Mountain Pose symmetrical stable energized standing pose

Tvacha Kriya: Dry Brushing the entire surface of the skin detox technique

Ujjayi breath: a pranayama; breath to quiet the senses and create focus in the mind

Utkatasana: an asana; Chair Pose

Utkatsana Sucirandhrasana: an asana; Cross-Legged Chair Pose

Uttanasana: an asana, Easy Forward Fold; easy forward fold with bent knees

Vairagya: non-attachment, surrender, or acceptance (oh well!)

Vinyasa: to place in a special way, movement skillfully on breath in a series

Viparita Karani: an asana; Legs Up the Wall Pose

Viradbhadrasana 2: an asana; Warrior 2 Standing Pose

Vrksasana: an asana; Tree Balance Pose

Further Reading

(a sampling, not a complete list)

The Relaxation Response by Dr. Herbert Bensen

Chakra Yoga by Alan Finger

Creative Visualization by Shakti Gawain

You Can Heal Your Life by Louise Hay

Eastern Body, Western Mind: Psychology and Chakra System as a Path to the Self, by Judith Anodea

Wheels of Life: User's Guide to the Chakra System by Judith Anodea

Anatomy of the Spirit: The Seven Stages of Power and Healing by Caroline Myss, Ph.D.

Women's Bodies, Women's Wisdom by Dr. Christiane Northrup

The Power of Positive Thinking by Dr. Norman Vincent Peale

Chakra Meditation by Swami Saradananda

A Women's Book of Yoga and Health by Sparrowe and Walden

Yoga of Heart; the Healing Power of Intimate Connection by Mark Whitwell

ॐ

In closing, I hope you are reading this after a delicious night's sleep, ready to start another intentionally healthy and joyful day. Thank yourself for practicing and don't hesitate to reach out to me at **melaniesalvatoreaugust.com** or others on the path of yoga (your local yoga studio) for more insights and support. You are not alone, and I am so happy that you have joined this sangha or family, the Love Tribe.

Acknowledgements

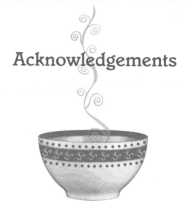

Thank you to Lisa McGuinness for believing in my abilities to create and for the positive and receptive space she established for me to share this practice. To Rose Wright, for her beautiful designs and pose depictions that we lovingly named (Ben, Satya and Lily). To my mother and father who always encouraged me to write and allowed me to read every "new age" book I could get my hands on (I still hold dear my tattered "creative visualization" by Shakti Gawain.) To my husband, Rafael August, who from the moment we came together was the key that unlocked my clarity and confidence to live my ideal life. To the teachers Amma, Alan Finger, Jean Koerner, Jenny Aurthur, Mark Whitwell, Elena Brower, Dr. Susan Taylor, Martin Rader, and Robert Francisconi, who have had such a positive influence on my life. To Mynx Inatsugu, Nikki Estrada, Lakshmi Angie Norwood, Jessica Boylston-Fagonde, Rachel Scott, Michelle Giancola, Amy Sui, and Christina Moore who have by example and endless discussions inspired me to deepen my own understanding of the process of connecting and communicating my dharmic purpose. To the "Love Tribe" whose love, energy, and support are instrumental in my understanding of the essence of what is transformative in this vast practice of yoga. To my deliciously wild little boys Giovanni, Casciato, and Roman, who played quietly (or not) beside me as I wrote this book, I love you with all of my being. A final special thank you to Joan Franciosa-August and Boyer P. August whose unconditional love and caretaking of said little boys on our La Dolce Terra enabled me to finish this manuscript on time.

To learn more about Melanie Salvatore-August and her inspirational practice check out **melaniesalvatoreaugust.com** where soon you will be able to download instructions for many of the poses found in *Kitchen Yoga*.